Introduction

This booklet gives you an introc ...y failure.

At the end you will find a 'jargon busting' section to help explain medical terms, and also a guide to further information in books and online.

Every person is different and has different treatment requirements; the booklet contains general advice only, and the treatment for each person's kidney failure must be decided on an individual basis.

Contents

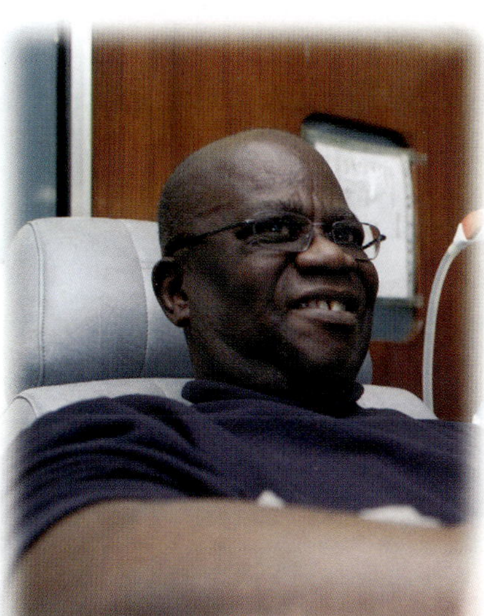

What is kidney failure?

About one in every ten people has some abnormality in the kidneys. Only a few people with kidney disease develop serious damage to their kidneys, which is called kidney failure. The term 'kidney failure' means that the kidneys are working at less than one third (30%) of normal.

The function of the kidneys may remain stable for many years, even if kidney failure is present. However, in many people the function of the kidneys slowly deteriorates. If the kidney function falls to less than one seventh (15%) of normal, kidney failure becomes life threatening.

Even with advanced kidney failure, the water that is passed as urine may look normal, but blood tests will show there is a build-up of chemicals in the blood that should have been eliminated by the kidneys.

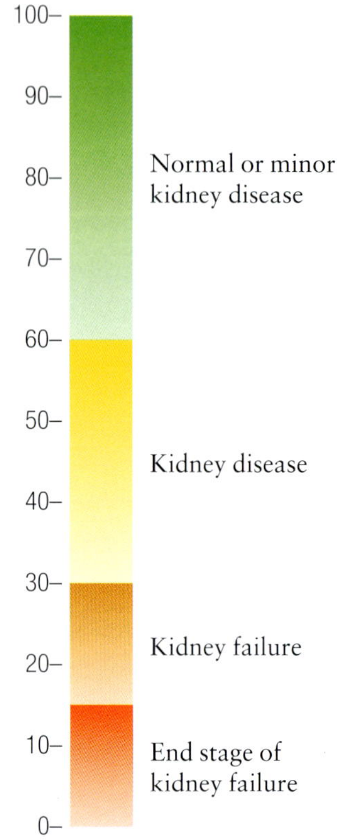

Some causes of kidney failure

- High blood pressure (often with hardening and narrowing of the arteries to the kidneys)
- Diabetes
- Inflammation in the kidneys (nephritis, or glomerulonephritis)
- Polycystic kidney disease

What happens to the body in kidney failure?

1. **Chemical build-up** The kidneys are meant to get rid of chemical waste from the body. In kidney failure the levels of these chemicals are too high. The body can often tolerate high levels of build-up without any symptoms, but eventually there will be tiredness, sickness, itching and anaemia.
2. **Fluid control** The kidneys control the amount of water in the body. In many people with kidney failure, the amount of fluid in the body continues to be controlled, but in others the kidneys may lose control and the body can contain too much or too little fluid.
3. **High blood pressure** The kidneys normally control the level of blood pressure in the body. The blood pressure is usually too high in kidney failure.

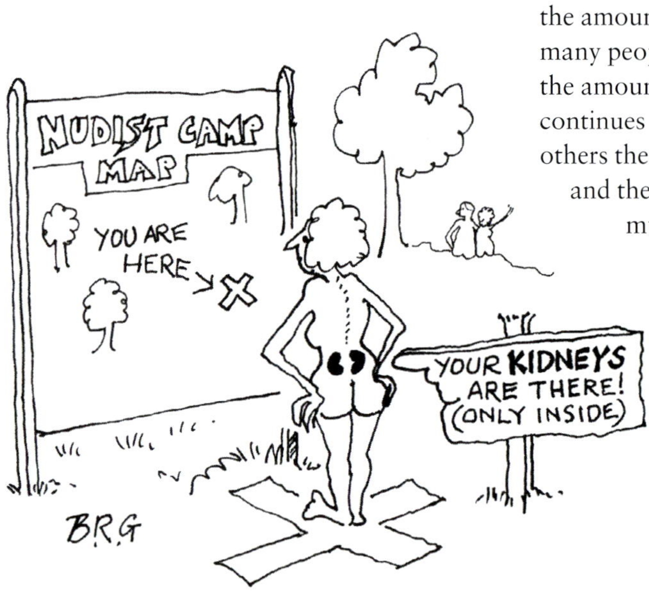

Treatment starts early

Treatment for kidney failure should start when the kidney function is down to about one third (30%) of normal. Most people do not feel ill at this stage, but the body is being affected in many ways. Dialysis or a transplant will be considered when the kidney function gets down to about one seventh (15%) of normal. It is best to start planning for this treatment well in advance because it takes some time to cope with the shock of developing such a serious illness, and there are several choices to make about the best type of treatment.

How to cope

Get the facts straight

It is important you understand what is going on inside your body. This book only provides general advice, so detailed information about each individual person and their needs must come from other sources, as in the box below.

Sources of information

People to talk to:

- Nurses
- Renal pharmacist
- Doctors
- Other patients
- Dietitians
- Renal social worker

Written information:

- Information leaflets available on the Renal Unit
- Books on renal failure
- Internet

Support groups:

- The local kidney patient association
- National kidney patient organisations
- Associations for different diseases (eg Diabetes UK)

See page 25 for further details

After being told that they have kidney failure, most people will feel shocked – as with other types of serious loss. It is totally normal to be upset and confused, and to try and deny what is happening.

Although kidney failure is stressful, people are resourceful. You may well find you have hidden strengths you never suspected. Although the experience can be dreadful at times, many people find it gives them a different outlook on life and they go on to feel better and stronger.

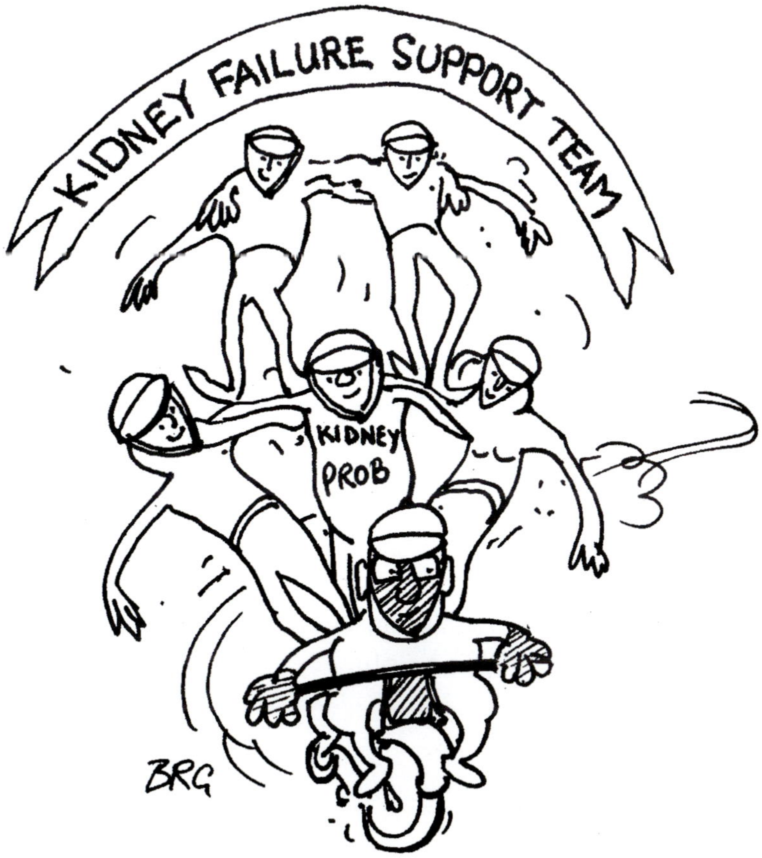

Get support

No-one can manage everything on their own – support from family, friends or hospital staff is absolutely essential. No-one wants to be a burden on anyone else, but hiding feelings from family and friends will make it more difficult in the long term. Support is a two way process, and no-one should feel guilty about asking for the type of emotional support they would be willing to offer others.

Key family members or friends are welcome to visit the Renal Unit, so they can understand what goes on.

If you think you may need help from the social services, or be entitled to financial allowances, talk to the social worker attached to your Renal Unit.

Coping strategies

People cope with kidney failure and have enormously successful lives, but it is not always easy and everyone has to overcome some problems from time to time. Every person does this in a different way, there is no 'formula' to make it easy.

Some coping strategies

- Have an activity to turn to for diversion (e.g. a hobby)
- Set goals (e.g. I will go to that wedding!)
- Keep up normal routines, even if you give up some sports or hobbies
- Learn to control disease, rather than being controlled by it

Trying to carry on as though absolutely nothing has happened causes more problems in the long term, and makes it harder to cope when anything goes wrong. It is necessary to recognise that kidney failure and dialysis are problems that will change your life.

As well as the nurses and doctors on the Renal Unit, the renal social worker can help with counselling, and some people find a professional psychologist helpful.

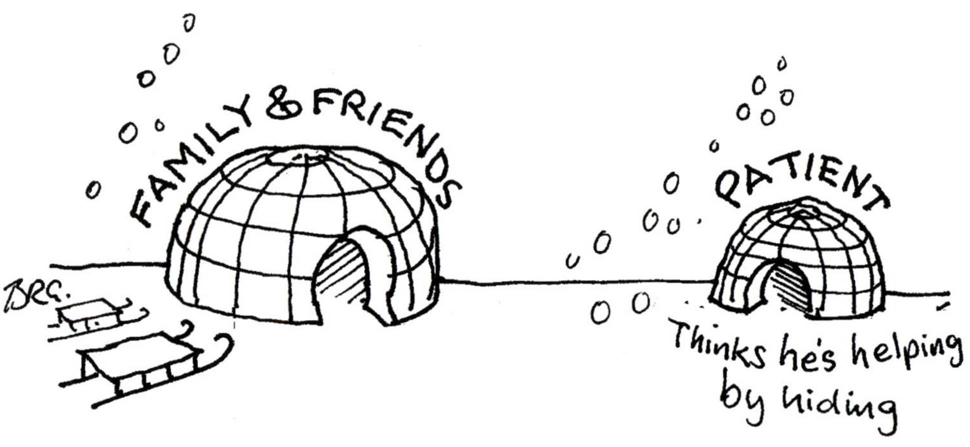

Maureen's story

The words 'you have kidney failure' are perhaps one of the most dreaded things you are going to hear. From that day forward you start a 'new life' of blood tests, diet and visits to a renal consultant who keeps you up to date with how your kidneys are functioning.

My first reactions were 'This isn't happening to me' and 'It will get better'. But of course it was, and it doesn't.

In my case there was a deterioration over years. The terrible tiredness and nausea were the most distressing, then the high blood pressure and finally I started to carry a lot of fluid. I got so exhausted and breathless that dialysis was the next step.

Now I had read about dialysis in a magazine and I for one wasn't having any part of that, thank you very much. But the dreaded day eventually arrived and I turned up at the Renal Unit very tired, breathless and scared. I was taken to the unit, the nurses explained what was going to happen and before I had time to think I was connected up. I was really surprised it wasn't anything like I had imagined. And when I came off, 'wonderful', I could really breathe properly again. Everyone was helpful and friendly.

Having kidney failure does not mean you need to stop enjoying life!

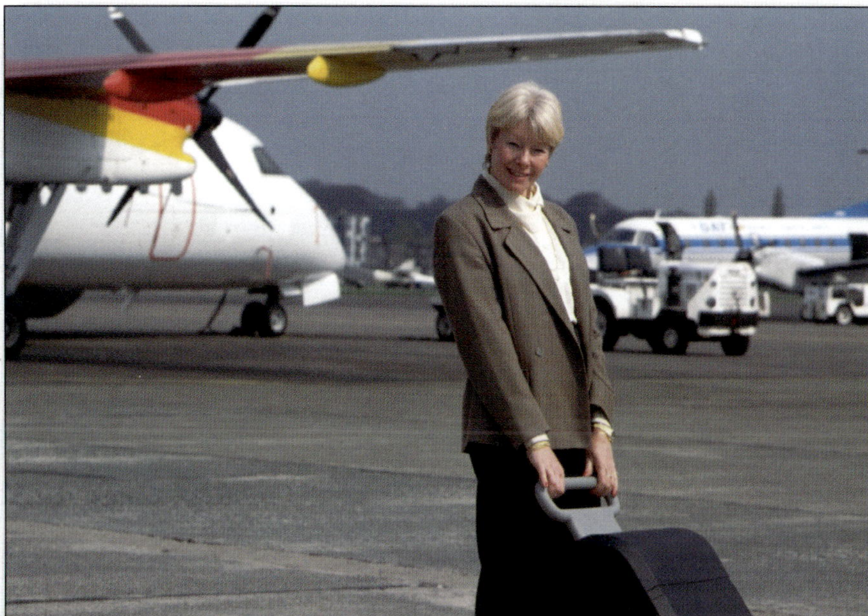

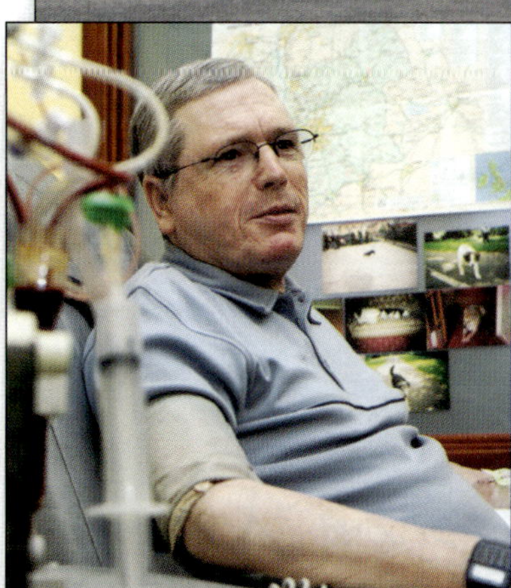

▲*You can take PD fluid, or even an APD machine, on holiday with you.*

◀ *Regular dialysis allows Stuart to get out with his beloved dogs.*

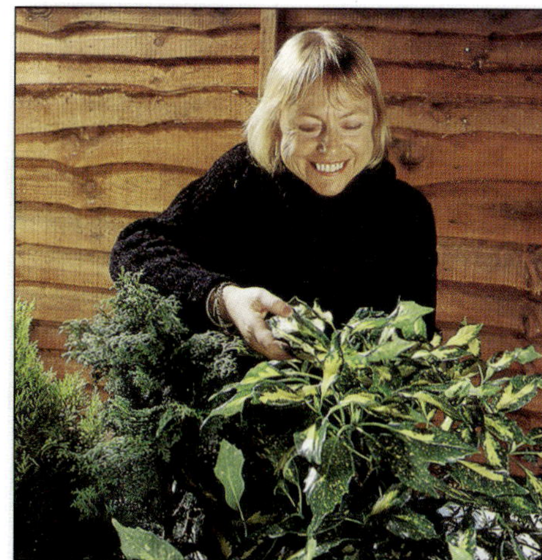

Gardening is a source of pleasure for many – with or without kidney failure.

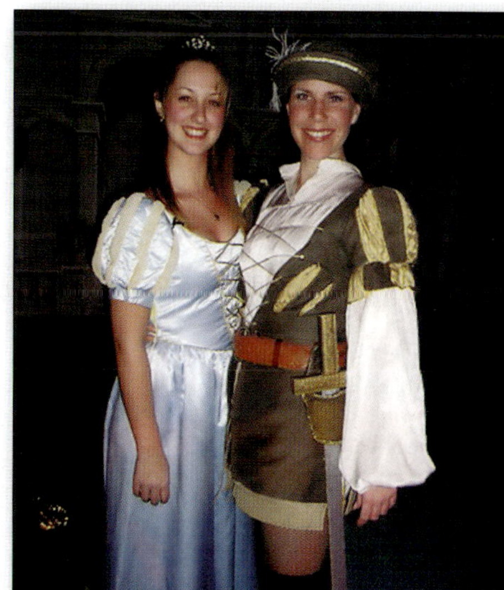

Nikki (on right) has a new kidney and can continue playing starring roles.

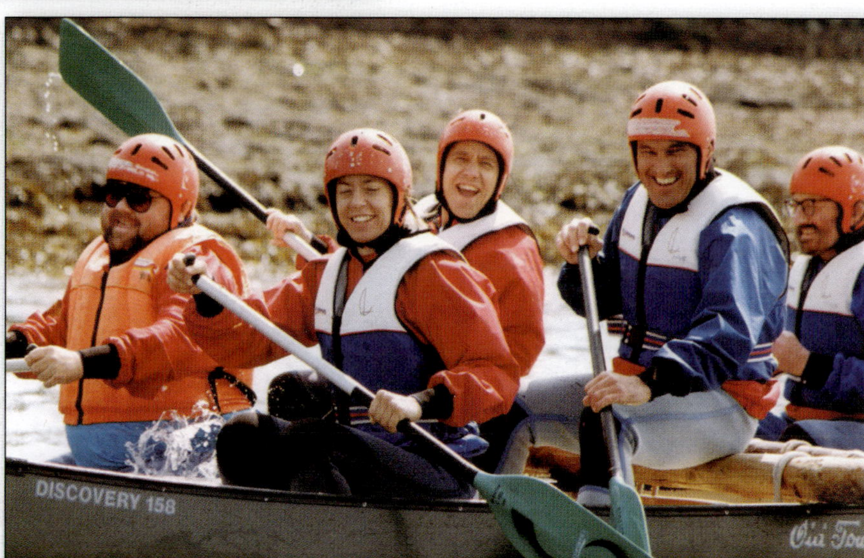

Even active sports, such as white water rafting, need not be given up.

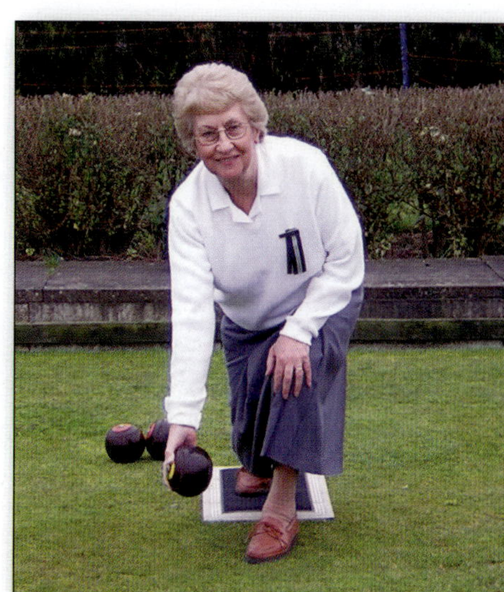

Vivienne enjoys the gentler, but no less competitive, world of bowls.

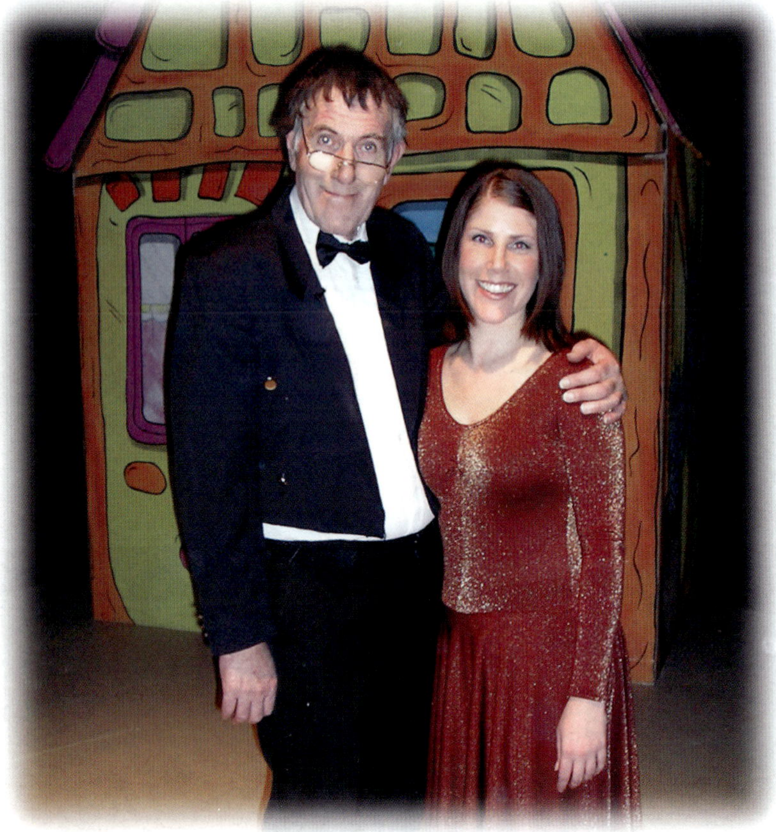

Nikki with her father, Graham, 'treading the boards' during one of their annual fundraising cabarets.

Nikki has a transplanted kidney, donated by Graham 9 years ago and is able to lead a full and active life, following her dreams.

Nikki's story

I can sympathise with anyone who has kidney failure, particularly young people.

I was diagnosed at age 20. I was a dancer, had just left stage school and taken all my major exams. I had lots of dreams and ambitions and felt that my life was just beginning. I ate really healthily and many people said I was the healthiest person they knew.

A month after I'd left college the bomb dropped. To cut a long story short, I ended up in hospital and after many tests was told what I'd got. I can't really express how I felt. Shock, numbness, confusion and a number of other emotions, but most of all an overwhelming feeling that my life and career were over before they'd begun.

The most difficult things to get through were choosing which type of dialysis to go on, and understanding the illness and why it all happens. With the great support of family, friends and the wonderful hospital staff I went onto CAPD [Continuous Ambulatory Peritoneal Dialysis] and gradually started to feel better, accept it all and try to get on with my life.

A year and a half later I had a transplant from my Dad, I now have my own dancing school and feel very fortunate. It is very easy to feel negative and feel down and upset but I think that all of this has made me a stronger person who doesn't have to take things for granted any more. And I always remember that there are people worse off than me.

Isambard's story

At first it was difficult to make the transition from being a fit and healthy person (so I thought) who can come and go at will, to becoming the focus of such oppressive concern at home. It almost drove me insane.

My family – very much involved in keeping me alive – also took time to get the measure of the illness. I met the disease at every turn: in my pills, in my diet, in bodily function, in my family's attitude, and in my limited ability to socialise. I was hemmed in. Just as initially I resented the idea of being dependent on medication for the rest of my life, so I resented my dependence on people around me for food, shelter and support.

A tremendous amount of support is required for kidney patients, especially through the dialysis and transplant process.

Kidney failure specialists – the Renal Unit

People with kidney failure see kidney specialists as well as the general practitioner. Nearly every city in the UK has a kidney unit, or visiting specialists who hold clinics in the local hospital. The kidney specialist team is usually based in the Renal Unit, 'renal' being another word for kidney.

It is important for each person to find out exactly who from the Renal Unit will be providing each aspect of their care, and write down a list of names and telephone numbers or email addresses. No single person, not even a doctor who is a kidney consultant, is an expert on everything.

It is also important to keep in touch with your general practitioner and local health centre. Your GP may not have expert knowledge about kidney failure, but he or she will know you and your health history better than the Renal Unit does, and can provide some monitoring closer to home than the hospital.

Your relationship with the specialist Renal Unit

What the Unit should do for you:

- Agree a plan of treatment with you, offering the right choices
- Provide information, including copies of clinic letters if you want them
- Provide clear contact details
- Respond to questions and complaints politely and honestly

What you should do for the Renal Unit:

- Cancel appointments for clinics or tests in advance if you can't attend
- Tell someone if you don't understand or agree with your treatment
- If you suffer from any allergies, make sure the staff know about them
- Read clinic letters and lists of medication to make sure there are no mistakes
- The Renal Unit is not perfect; help correct mistakes politely

Some members of the Renal Unit team

Consultant
Senior doctor (you may see several consultants)

Pre-dialysis nurse
Nurse specialising in kidney failure

Renal dietitian
Will advise on suitable diet

Renal pharmacist
Will advise on medication

Renal social worker
A social worker attached to the unit

Anaemia (or EPO) nurse
Will advise on the prevention and treatment of anaemia

Transplant coordinator
The person responsible for organising transplant listing and work-up

This is only a guide; renal units differ slightly, so check out local facilities

Isambard's story

In renal units, one sees people who have had all manner of complications from an early age, such as people with diabetes who have had amputations. Most of them are not putting on brave faces, but in fact have a genuine reserve of cheerfulness.

In this place of extremes I found what lay ahead worrying at first. But then, seeing how others managed, I found it easier to understand my own predicament.

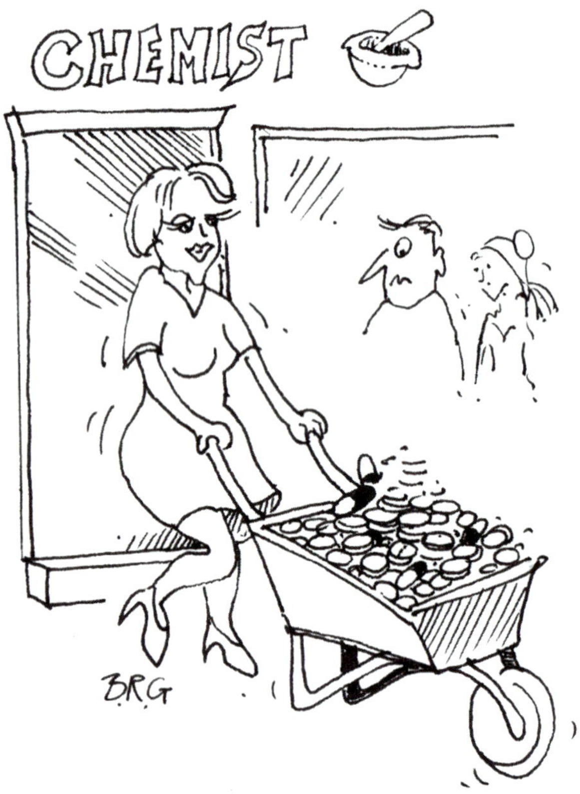

Medical treatment of kidney failure

Before dialysis or a transplant is required, the effects of kidney failure need treatment. This can be by:

- Blood tests and drugs
- Diet
- Controlling fluid balance
- Controlling blood pressure
- Combatting anaemia

Blood tests and drugs

Blood tests are required at regular intervals. Many of the problems that develop in kidney failure do not cause any symptoms until a late stage, so blood tests are important to detect abnormalities early.

The most important blood test is 'creatinine', which measures kidney function. A normal level is about 100 µmol/l, kidney failure is significant when it goes up to 250-300 µmol/l, and dialysis is needed at about 500-700 µmol/l. The creatinine may be converted to a measurement of renal function called 'clearance', or GFR (glomerular filtration rate). Normal is about 100 ml/min, or down to 60 ml/min in older people. Kidney failure is significant when the level is 30 ml/min, and dialysis is considered when the level is 10-15 ml/min.

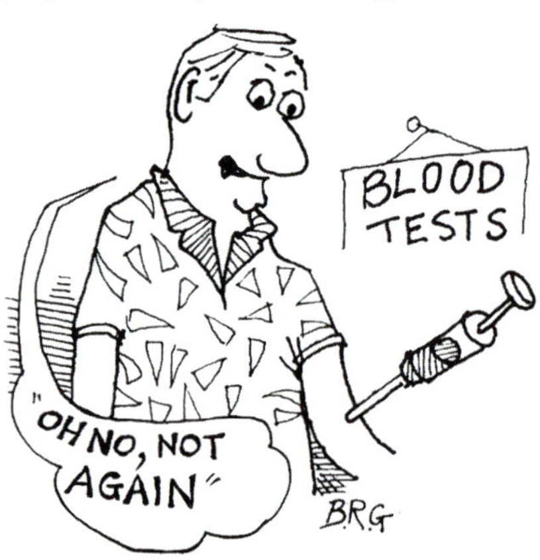

For each routine clinic visit a range of tests are requested, including 'bone' and 'liver' tests – these are routine and do not mean the bones and liver necessarily have any problems. Before dialysis and transplantation are started, tests are required for viral hepatitis and HIV (the AIDS virus).

Several different types of tablet and other medications are required by most people with kidney failure. It is not unusual for ten different types of tablet to be prescribed, each doing a different job. These can be very effective in controlling the effects of kidney failure, but it is also very important to understand the 'golden rules' (in the box on the right), and to get into the habit of taking them regularly and at the right times.

Golden rules about tablets and other medications

1. Carry a list of all medications, and check with the hospital and your GP that the list is correct
2. When a new drug is started:
   - understand why it is being given
   - find out what side effects might occur
   - make sure it does not react with any of the other treatment being given
3. If any side effects develop, ask a doctor or the Renal Pharmacist for advice
4. Don't stop medication without telling anyone
5. Store all tablets in their original containers, in a cool dry place out of the reach of children
6. Only remove tablets from the bottle/box when it is time to take them
7. Order new supplies of tablets in good time:
   - most tablets are prescribed by the GP, some may come from the hospital

Fluid balance

There is a large amount of fluid (water) in the body, which must be kept at the right level. Normally the kidneys control the fluid level, but this control is lost in many people with kidney failure, and in nearly everyone receiving dialysis.

If there is too much fluid in your body, some will collect around your ankles or in your lungs. Fluid in the lungs causes breathlessness. Extra fluid can cause very high blood pressure, because the blood vessels have to expand to hold it (like blown up balloons).

If there is too little fluid in your body, the blood pressure can fall. This can cause you to feel dizzy or faint when standing up or trying to walk fast.

What is the 'fluid restriction'?

This is the maximum amount of fluid that can be taken each day. The restriction depends on how much fluid comes out, either through the kidneys, or with the dialysis machine. The Renal Unit will advise on the exact restriction. It is usually necessary to reduce salt intake as well as fluid intake.

Fluid conversions

Standard cup	180 mls
Half cup	90 mls
Full glass or coffee mug	200 mls
Half glass	100 mls
Milk with cereals	100 mls
Soup	100 mls
Cans/bottles	As marked

How much I have drunk?

Add up the amount of fluid taken each day. Fluid includes all types of watery drinks and food such as soup or gravy. Anything that is wet counts as fluid. Ice cubes also count as fluid, because they melt inside!

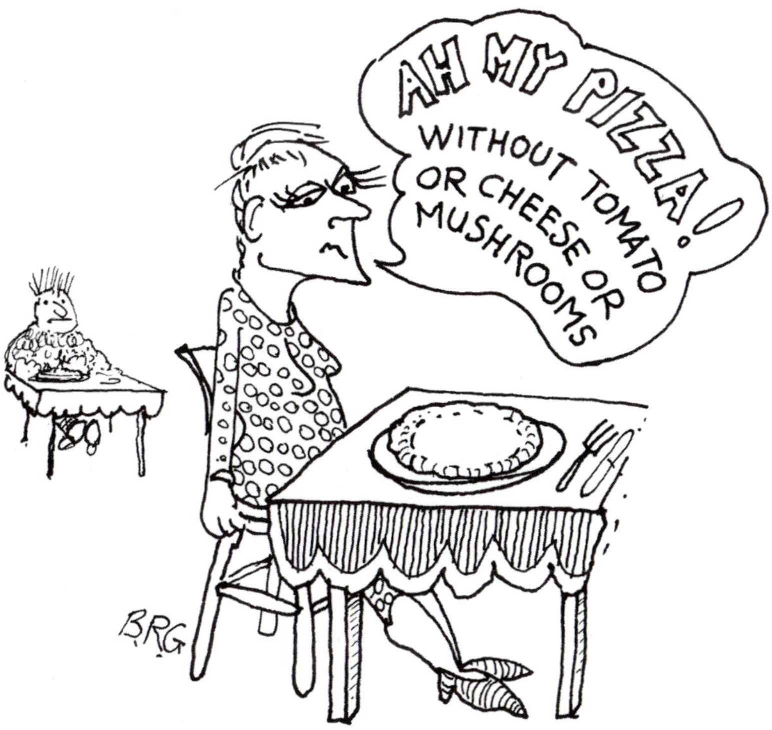

AH MY PIZZA!
WITHOUT TOMATO OR CHEESE OR MUSHROOMS
BRG

Diet

Because the kidneys eliminate waste products, when they don't work properly the diet needs to be modified. Taking the wrong diet could be very serious. Diet in kidney failure is not just about reducing the intake of certain foods. It is important to keep enjoying eating, and to eat well because poor nutrition can also cause problems. A good diet can delay dialysis for some time. Even if you are on dialysis, it is very important for your general health to keep to an appropriate diet.

In advanced kidney failure dietary advice will be given by a specialist dietitian. A kidney failure diet is tailored to the individual, but should be balanced and healthy, usually with a reduced intake of salt, and often a reduced intake of two important minerals, potassium (coffee, bananas, crisps and tomatoes are high in potassium) and phosphate (milk, eggs and cheese are high in phosphate).

Managing your diet

- Talk to a dietitian before altering diet
- Diet should be healthy and balanced
- Most people should reduce salt intake

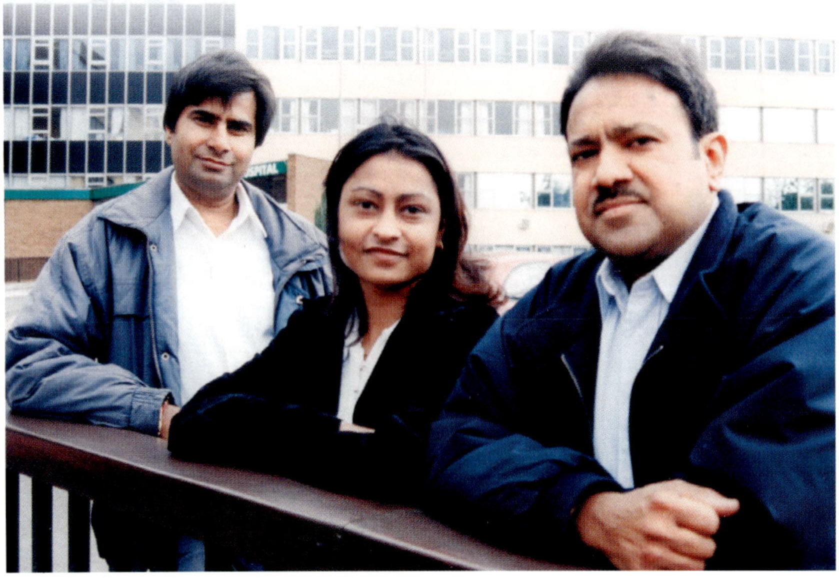

Unfortunately, kidney disease is common in people of South Asian descent, but Chod, Wendy and Nandlal cope well with dialysis.

Anaemia

Many people with kidney failure have a condition called anaemia. This means that they have a lack of red blood cells in their body.

Blood is made up of a liquid part and small particles called cells. Red cells carry oxygen around the body. Measuring the level of a substance called haemoglobin in the blood gives a guide to the number of red cells and whether a person is anaemic. (The level of haemoglobin in the blood is measured in g/dl, and the normal level is 12 g/dl or higher.)

The kidneys normally manage the production of red blood cells by making a hormone called erythropoietin (EPO). If you have kidney failure, your body will not be able to produce as much EPO and this will cause you to become anaemic.

However, you can now be given the drug EPO, which is an artificial version of natural EPO and can boost the body to make red blood cells. EPO is taken by about 1 in 5 (20%) people with advanced kidney failure, and about 2 in 3 (67%) people on dialysis.

A number of different companies make this artificial version of EPO, which needs to be given by injection. Most people soon learn how to inject themselves. EPO is available in a number of forms, for example pre-filled 'pens' or 'vials'.

The dose of EPO required varies from person to person according to the level of haemoglobin in your blood. Each injection only lasts for a period of time, and your likelihood of becoming anaemic won't reduce unless you have a successful transplant operation.

EPO may cause your blood pressure to rise especially at the beginning of treatment. It is important that the blood pressure is monitored.

As well as EPO, your body will also need iron and some vitamins if it is to produce haemoglobin. Many people need to take iron tablets as well as EPO. If iron tablets don't work, or cause side effects such as tummy pain, iron can be given through a drip in the arm.

Blood pressure

Blood flows around the body under pressure generated by the pumping action of the heart. The exact level of blood pressure can be measured from the pulse in the arm. If there are kidney problems it is common to have high blood pressure, and this puts strain on all the blood vessels in the body. This can make the kidneys fail faster, damage the heart and cause strokes. Sometimes high blood pressure can cause headaches, but usually you feel nothing.

The blood pressure varies from minute to minute according to activity and stress levels, and sometimes shoots up when people walk into in hospital clinics or GP surgeries. The blood pressure can be measured at home using machines bought from pharmacies and medical supplies companies. Those that measure the blood pressure from a cuff around the upper arm are the most reliable. If you measure your blood pressure at home using one of these devices, this will give your doctor particularly useful information about your blood pressure. However, you must remember to have the device regularly serviced and calibrated to check that it is accurate.

Tablets are often necessary to control the blood pressure, and many people find they need several types. It is important to take blood pressure tablets regularly, but do speak up if there are any side effects, as it is usually possible to change to another type of tablet.

What is the ideal blood pressure?

Blood pressure is measured by two numbers. These give the highest pressure the heart pumps blood out at, and the lowest pressure in the artery between heartbeats. An ideal blood pressure would be less than 130/80 mmHg. However, this is not achievable in everyone, especially older people who may have some hardening of the arteries.

Choices about dialysis and transplantation

Every person with advanced kidney failure needs to make some choices about the type of treatment that is best for them. It is best to plan in advance. Putting off decisions until the last minute may mean more complications or a longer spell in hospital than is necessary.

Planning in advance does mean making choices about major medical treatments before kidney failure causes ill health. Information, support and having time to make the best choices will be enormously helpful.

◆ No dialysis – 'conservative' treatment

Dialysis can put strain on the body and may lead to complications, or even death. For some people who have severe disease in other parts of their body, it may be best not to have dialysis. Although this means the person will eventually die of kidney failure, if the deterioration of the kidneys is slow, it may be possible to live for months or a couple of years. It may not be possible to be as active or as fit as with good dialysis, but this may not matter if someone's lifestyle is limited by other health problems. Management without dialysis is called 'conservative' treatment.

Most people who opt to have conservative treatment are aged over 75 years. However, suitability for dialysis is not determined by age, and many people in their 80s who are otherwise fit have enormously successful lives on dialysis.

It is unusual for people under the age of 70 to choose conservative treatment, but this approach may be appropriate for people with very serious heart disease or other problems. Additionally, no-one is compelled to have dialysis and can choose not to have the treatment, however medically suitable they may be for dialysis.

Conservative treatment requires ongoing medical input to help control symptoms and regulate the diet. Particularly important is the treatment of anaemia with EPO injections (see previous page), which can be effective in getting rid of some tiredness, itching and loss of appetite.

Death from kidney failure is not normally painful. Most people become weak and eventually pass into a coma. Feelings of agitation and sickness can be treated with drugs, and care may be given at home or in hospital. Many kidney units are developing links with hospices and other services to provide support and care during the terminal stages of kidney failure.

Treatment choices in kidney failure

◆ No dialysis

'Conservative' treatment – may suit people with other medical problems and slowly progressive kidney failure

◆ Kidney transplant

The best treatment for kidney failure in people fit enough for the operation. The best type of transplant, if possible, is from a living donor, given just before dialysis is needed

◆ Haemodialysis

Blood is washed through a machine. Can be given in hospital as an outpatient, in a local 'satellite' unit, or at home

◆ Peritoneal dialysis

Uses a tube in the tummy. Fluid is passed in and out of the tummy four times a day at home, or overnight at home using a machine

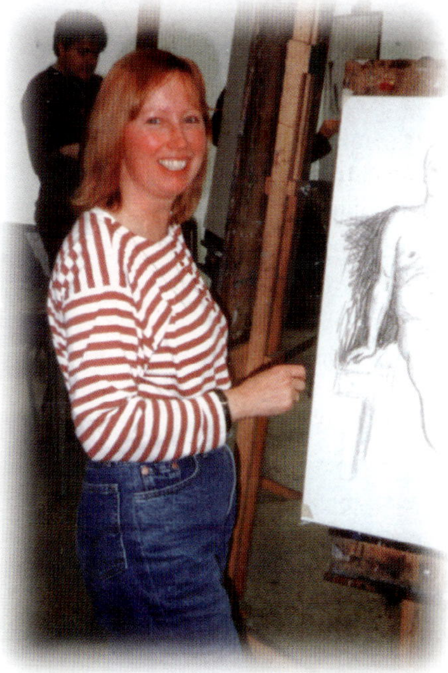

Grace chose home haemodialysis to give her the flexibility she needed while studying art. She went on to have a successful transplant.

◆ Kidney transplantation

Successful kidney transplantation is the best treatment for kidney failure. However it is not a complete cure. Someone else's kidney will not work 100% after being transplanted, and transplants do not function for ever. It is necessary to take drugs every day to stop your body from 'rejecting' the new kidney, but transplants still sometimes fail despite this. However the quality of life is likely to be much better with a good transplant than on dialysis.

If you have heart disease, or a recent history of cancer, it may not be safe to have a transplant. Each person will be assessed by their medical team.

The best results for kidney transplants are achieved by having a transplant from a living donor, given just before dialysis is necessary. Current results show that 19 out of 20 (95%) transplanted kidneys are still working at the end of the first year, and the average survival of the transplant is about 15 years.

It takes months to organise a kidney transplant from a living donor, so planning in advance is necessary. A donor must be very healthy. A history of heart attack, cancer or other serious illness may rule out donation. As well as the medical tests, the donor and the recipient will be given plenty of information by the transplant coordinator, so that everyone has full understanding of all the issues. For good reasons, it is illegal to 'buy' a kidney from someone, or pay them for donating it. However, the law also recognises that giving an organ for transplant involves surgery, recovery time and often considerable absence from work. So financial support should be available for a donor who loses earnings or incurs other necessary expenses.

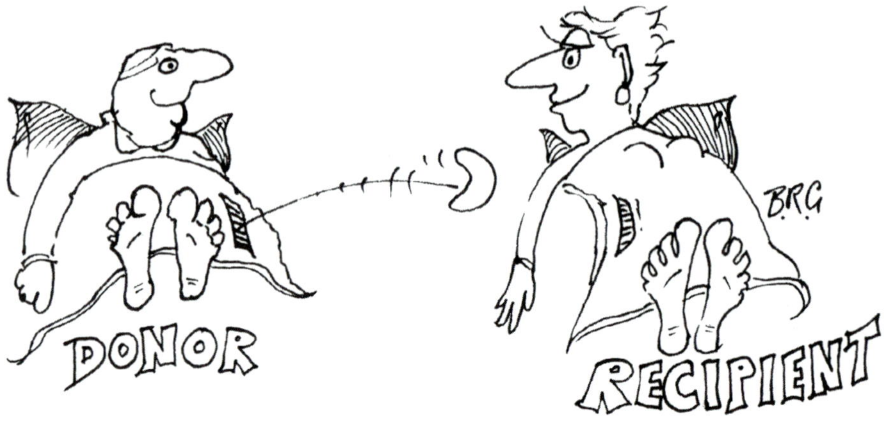

If a suitable living kidney donor is not available, your name will be placed on a list to wait for a kidney taken from someone who has died. There is a shortage of transplants from deceased donors, so although it is possible to put some people on the transplant list just before starting dialysis, there is usually a long wait for a transplant.

The transplant list is not a strict waiting list; kidneys are allocated according to blood group and tissue type. Therefore anyone on the list could get a kidney at any time. Nine out of ten (90%) kidneys taken from deceased donors will be working one year after transplantation, and on average they will continue to work for another 12-15 years.

Isambard had a transplant from a deceased donor

The call for a transplant came at 2.30 a.m. eight months after I had started on dialysis. I did not really feel in the mood for a major operation and, although trying to share the transplant co-ordinator's sense of joy on the telephone, I was terrified. I left within half an hour.

Now, over a year after the operation, all is going smoothly. With only the pills to take daily and three monthly check-ups, life has changed beyond all recognition.

The feeling of well-being, both physical and psychological, is astounding. More energised, healthier, and freed from the shackles of dialysis, I feel human again. A day does not pass without feeling gratitude towards the donor's family.

I can only hope that it might be of some minor consolation to them that the transplant has given me the opportunity to lead a full and unfettered life once more. A miraculous second chance.

Pam became a 'living kidney donor'

Would I still say 'Yes'?

Absolutely. Although I am not sure that I ever made such a conscious decision. It was more a series of small steps which eventually led to the day when two teams of skilled medical staff removed my left kidney and transplanted it into my brother.

I spoke to my family and arranged to have the first of a series of tests to determine the level of compatibility. No-one willingly undertakes a major operation without some misgivings. I remember feeling frustrated at how little information was available about the procedure, even though I was assured of the routine nature of the exercise.

Once the issue of compatibility had been resolved the Team then focused on my own kidneys. What was their 'plumbing' like? Which one would be the easiest to remove? Were they both in good condition? More 'Yes's'.

Then there were further consultations with both clinical and psychological specialists. How would I have felt had the operation proceeded, but failed? Not very happy, but the question had to be asked and answered.
Another 'Yes'?

The final rush to the actual operation is something for which you cannot really prepare. The calm professionalism of the medical staff is a valuable stabiliser.

I am not sure that I can recall the few days immediately after the operation. It is a major procedure and there are a few missing days in my life. My family and the nursing staff kept me comfortable and in no time at all my brother was trundling his drips into my ward!

Now, six months on, I am still aware that I underwent surgery and that it may take a few more months to return to my original fitness level. But I only have to see my brother fit and well and able to contribute to his family life to know that I made the right decision. The worry I had over my brother's ill health and discomfort has been replaced with a deep sense of satisfaction that I have been able to help him to overcome that sort of circumstance.

And yes, I would still say 'Yes'.

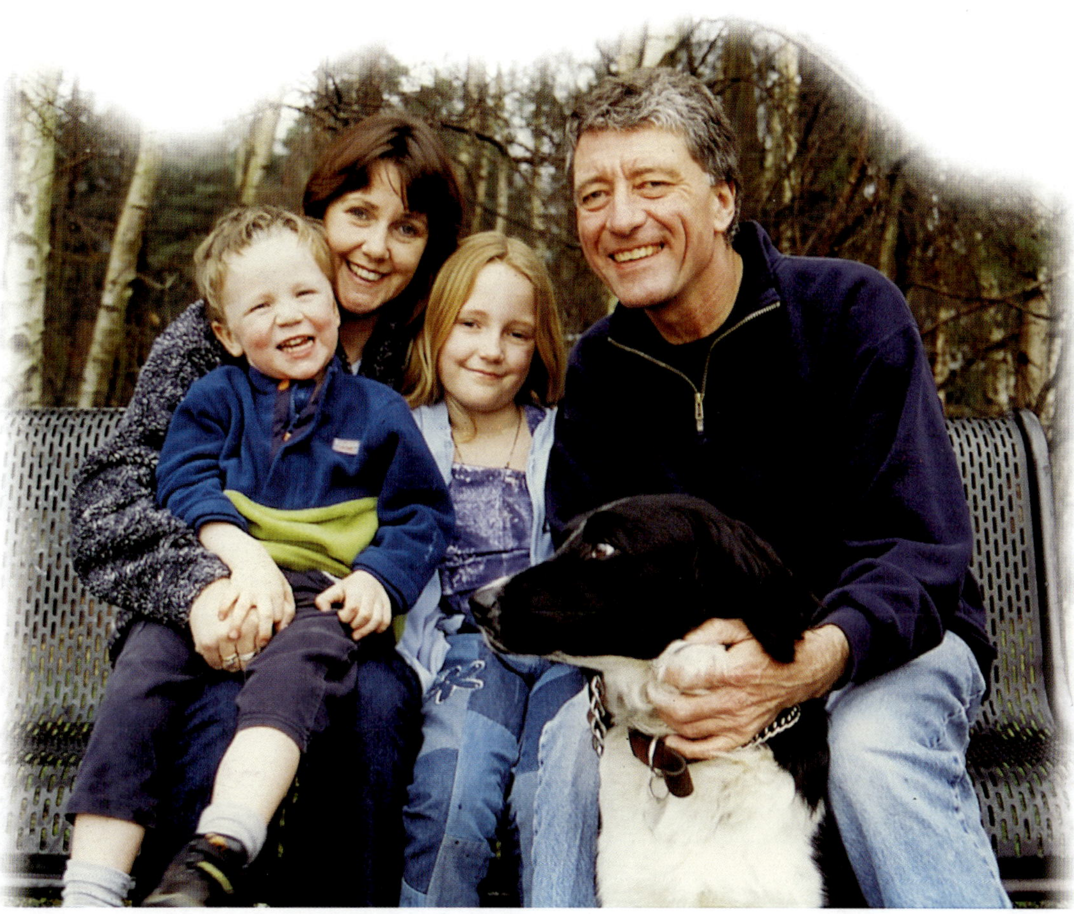

◆ Peritoneal dialysis (PD) *See also pages 16-17*

A plastic tube is inserted into your tummy, just below the belly button, by a small operation. The tube passes into your abdominal cavity (the peritoneum) and makes it possible for special fluid to be passed in and out of your tummy. The fluid is provided in plastic bags with tubing, and it is necessary to connect and disconnect the tubes. The fluid absorbs impurities from the blood, so cleaning your body. Changing the bag has to be done very carefully to avoid infection.

There are two main types of PD. One of these, called CAPD (continuous ambulatory peritoneal dialysis), involves four bag changes a day. It takes about 20 minutes to change bags. The other type is called APD (automated peritoneal dialysis). A machine makes the changes overnight, but this does mean being attached to the machine continuously every night.

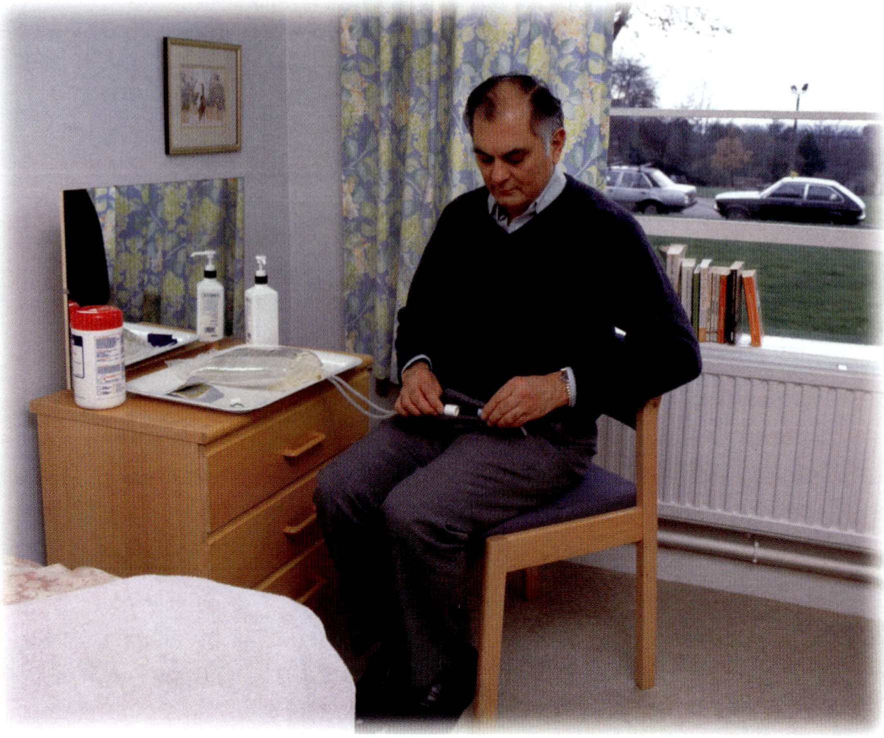

Many people find PD gives them a sense of control.

Isambard chose CAPD

In my case, the CAPD option offered independence from hospitals, and less in the way of fluid restrictions. A permanent line was inserted into my tummy, and I was taught the rigorous sterilisation techniques that accompany each exchange of dialysis fluid.

By the time I got home, boxes of dialysis bags had already arrived complete with all the attendant paraphernalia of iodine, dressings and sterilising fluid.

It took about five months to get the hang of dialysis. The morning rigmarole of changing the dressing on the catheter exit site, sterilising everything and then doing an exchange makes getting up a long-drawnout process.

Thus, suffering from what they call in the business 'problems of self-image', I returned with trepidation back into the pool of sexual activity. My first experience, however, gave me a rare insight into middle age: trying to make love with a protruding stomach, shortness of breath and a defective erection. Thankfully things did get better.

There were two bouts of peritonitis (an infection – due to my sloppiness in sterilising the area where I was doing exchanges – that causes stomach cramps and vomiting) which resulted in a dressing-down from the consultant.

At times there was a feeling of entrapment; for example, waking up at night and feeling perpetually connected to dialysis bags. When I tired of giving myself pep talks, or relapsed from focusing on the good things in life, from time to time a wave of sadness seized me.

The best experience for me, psychologically, was when I returned to work for two weeks in London (one of the marvels of the organisation that supplies the dialysis equipment is that, given enough time, it can deliver world-wide) and discovered that I could cope with doing dialysis at work.

What is dialysis?

Dialysis is also called 'artificial kidney treatment' as it replaces the function of the kidneys. It does not make the diseased kidneys work any better – these are normally left in place inside the body where they gradually lose all remaining function and shrivel up.

Dialysis does not replace the kidney function entirely. Some people feel almost back to normal on dialysis, most people are a bit limited, and a few people feel unwell on dialysis most of the time. If you are one of the unlucky ones who feels unwell most of the time, or has other complications, it is likely you will be able to change the type of dialysis, giving you the possibility of improving the outcome.

When should dialysis be started?

The symptoms of severe kidney failure are itching, vomiting and loss of appetite, or water retention with fluid on the lungs causing breathlessness. Dialysis should be started before these symptoms become severe. Blood tests give a guide to the severity of kidney failure, and are usually checked every 2-3 months. Dialysis is usually started when the blood creatinine level is about 500-700 μmol/l, compared to a normal level of about 100 μmol/l. Some specialists also refer to the 'clearance' or GFR, starting dialysis at a level of 10- 15 ml/min, compared to normal of about 100 ml/min. If your kidneys are deteriorating at a steady rate, it may be possible to predict in advance when the clearance will drop to a critical level.

Maureen's story: *Starting dialysis*

So now I've entered another stage of my life. 'Dialysis and me'. I am now on a different diet, as I'm allowed to eat more protein because the machine does some of the work of my kidneys. I receive my treatment and meet lots of other people with the same problems as myself. We talk and swap news and have a laugh.

The machine is my lifeline and because of it I am reasonably well and lead a good life, certainly a lot better than I did before I received dialysis, and I look healthier too.

◆ Haemodialysis

See also page 18

Haemodialysis involves blood being washed through a plastic 'artificial kidney' by a machine. This takes 3-4 hours, three times a week. The machine needs to get blood out of the body and to return it. This is done by means of needles in a 'fistula' in the arm, or by a plastic tube in the neck or under the collar bone. A 'fistula' is a swollen vein produced by a small operation on the arm.

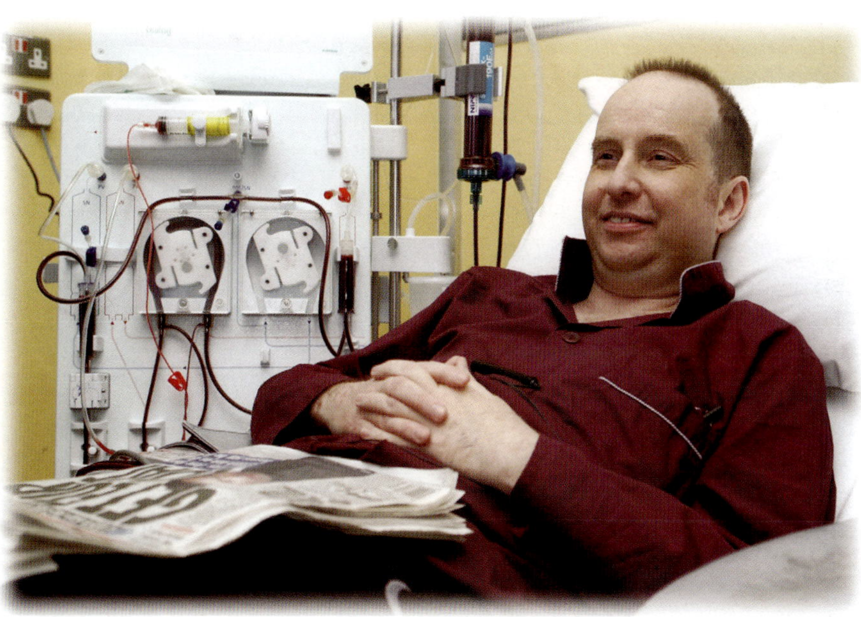

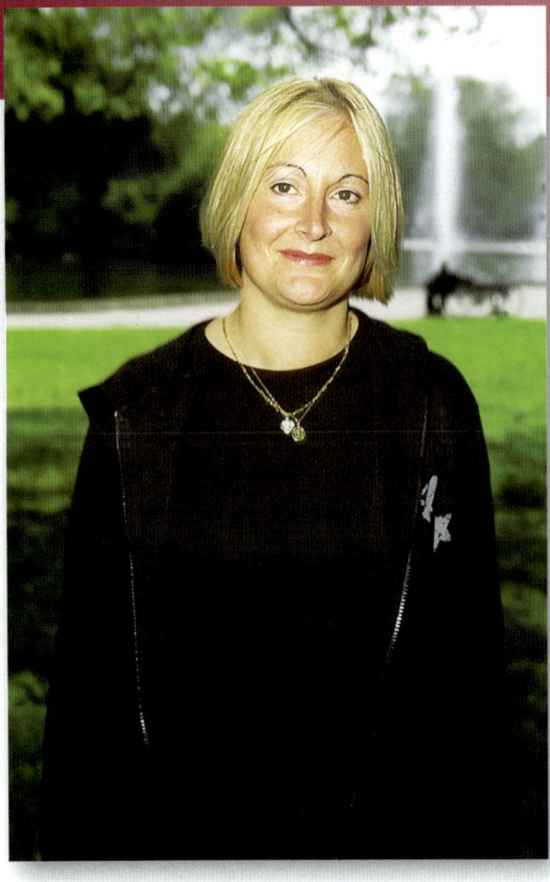

1 **This is Joanne who has been on CAPD since 1999.** *She will demonstrate how she does a CAPD exchange. These are normally done 4 times each day and take about 30-40 minutes. Please note that there is more than one type of CAPD connection on the market and they are different in detail, although in general the process is the same.*

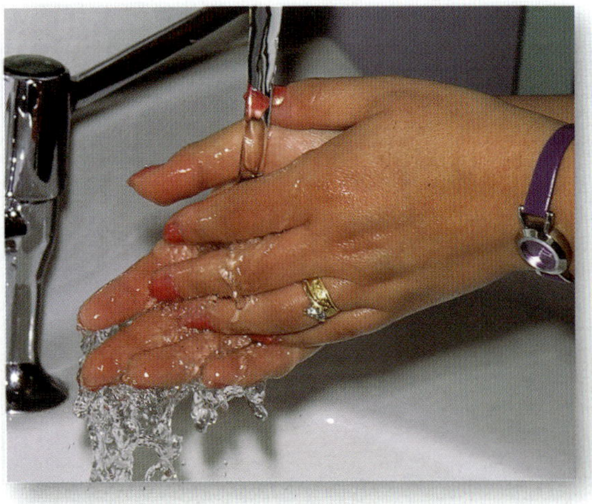

2 *In order to prevent the introduction of an infection during the CAPD exchange, Joanne washes her hands with a surgical scrub...*

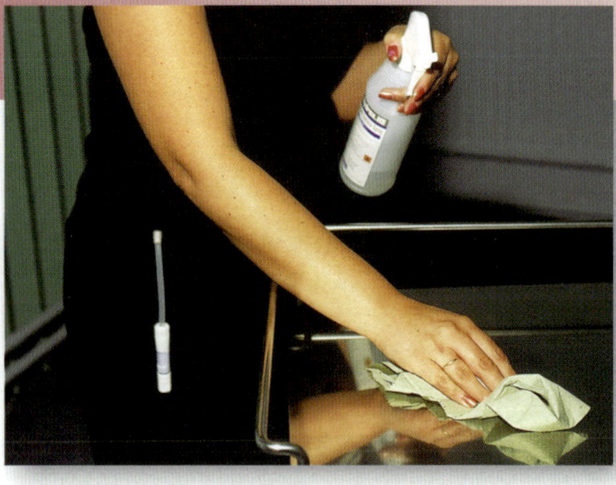

3 *...and also washes down the hard surface that will be used for the CAPD exchange.*

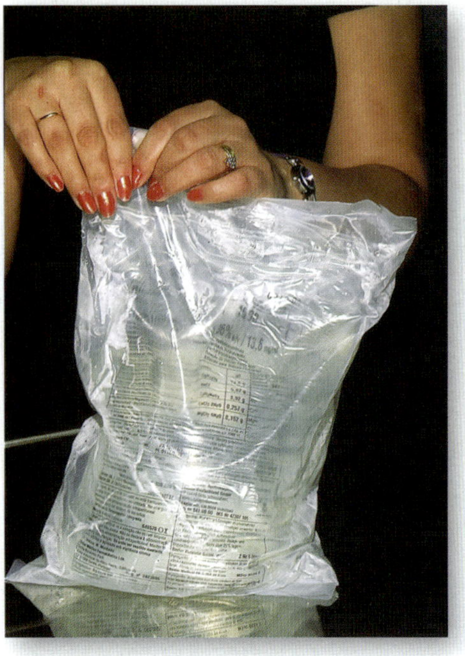

4 *The new bag of PD fluid comes with an empty bag into which the old dialysis fluid (that has been in the body since the last exchange) can be drained. Joanne opens the new bag, placing it on the cleaned surface.*

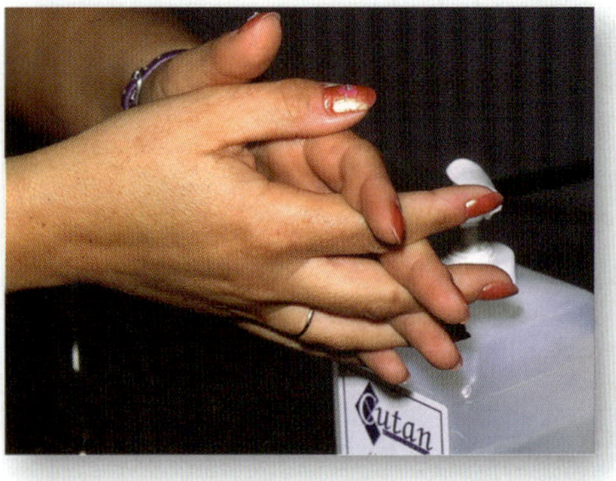

5 *Joanne now rubs her hands with a surgical alcohol solution. This ensures they are thoroughly clean before she connects the bag for her exchange.*

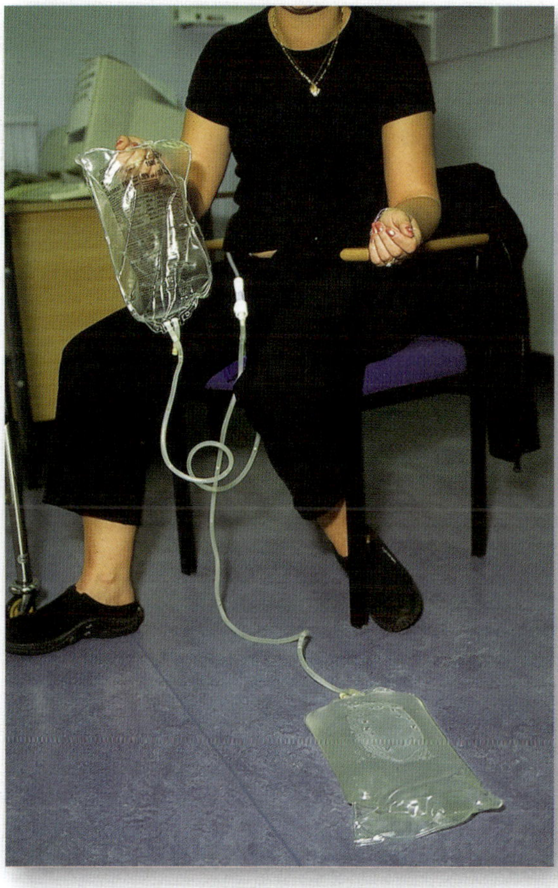

6 Joanne then carefully joins her catheter line up with the empty bag. She waits for 10-20 minutes while the old dialyis fluid drains from her tummy into the bag (on the floor). When the fluid has finished draining out, she checks that it is clear – any cloudiness could indicate an infection such as peritonitis. If Joanne sees this, she would need to contact her doctor without delay. After this, Joanne hangs up the new bag of dialysis fluid, connects it her catheter line, and lets it drain into her tummy. This usually takes about 5 minutes.

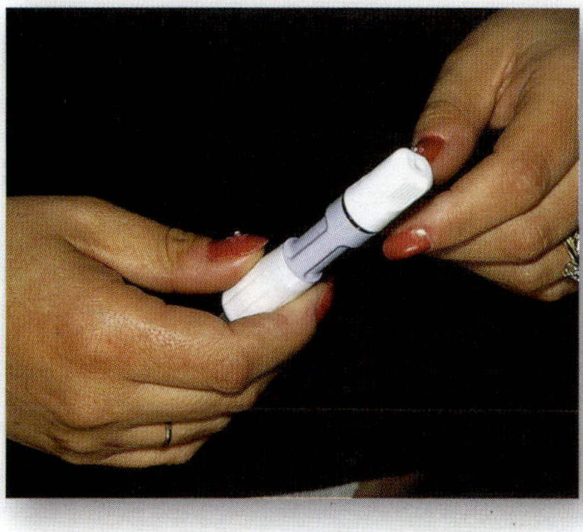

7 A disconnection cap is screwed onto the end of the catheter to keep the inside of the connection sterile until the next exchange.

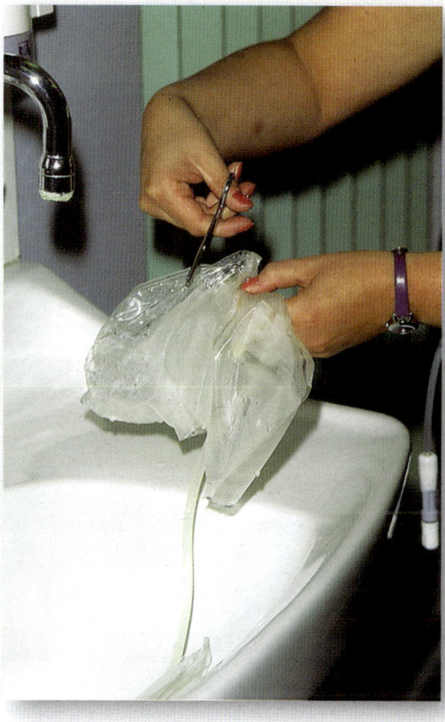

8 The bag containing the old dialysis fluid is cut and the fluid drained into the sink.

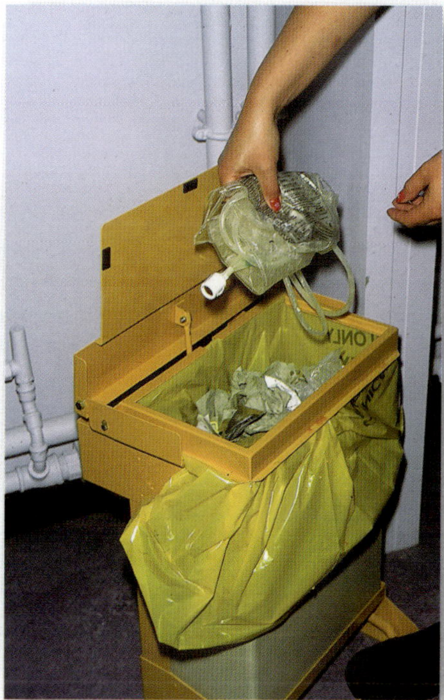

9 Joanne disposes of the old (empty) bag and lines in a medical waste sack which will go for incineration.

Haemodialysis

This is Patricia who has been on haemodialysis for several years.

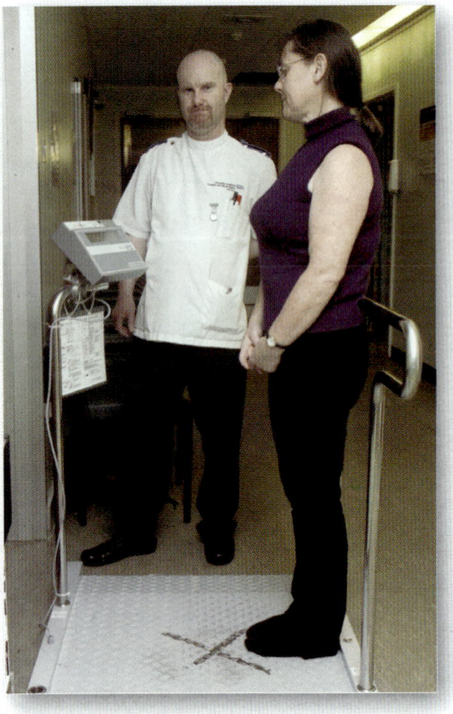

1 On arrival in the Unit, Patricia is weighed, to measure the amount of fluid that needs to be removed by the machine.

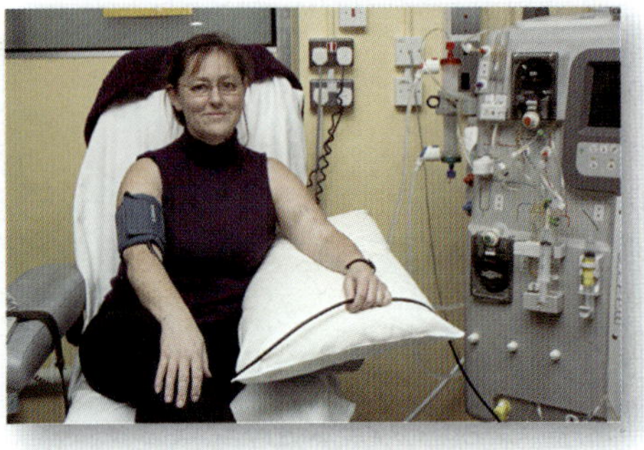

2 She sits in a reclining chair by the dialysis machine.

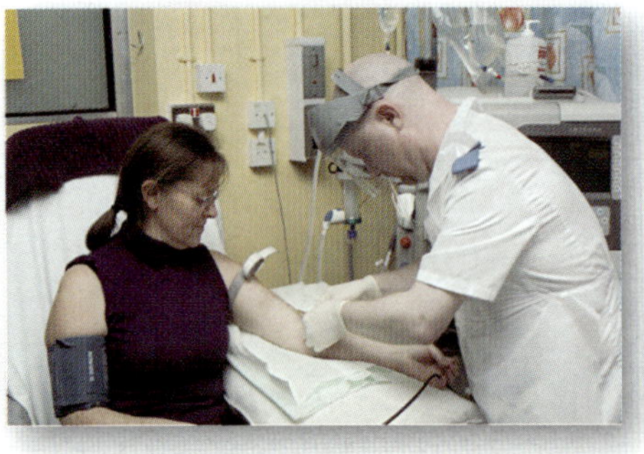

3 Needles are inserted into the dialysis 'fistula' in her arm.

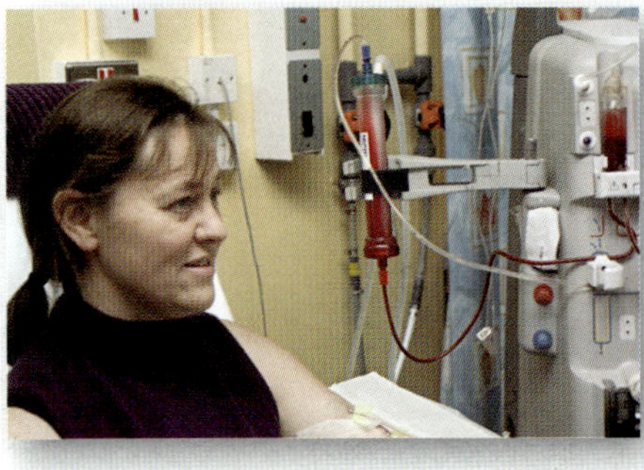

4 Blood is pumped through the machine – this is painless.

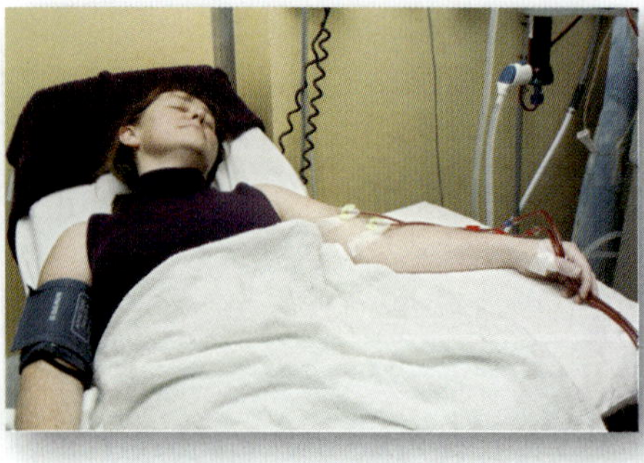

5 Her treatment lasts 4 hours. She sleeps for some of the time.

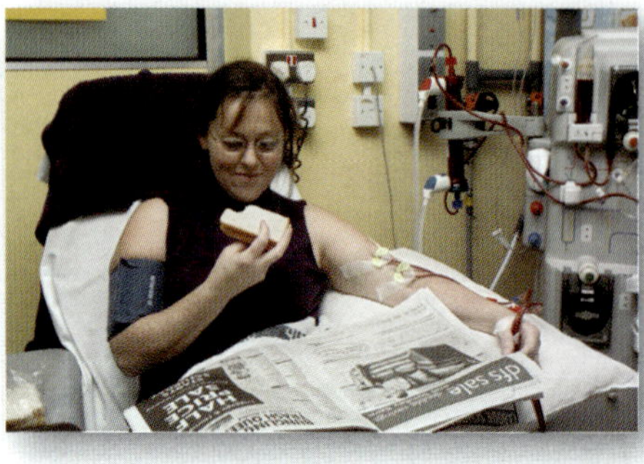

6 Patricia can also read and have a light snack.

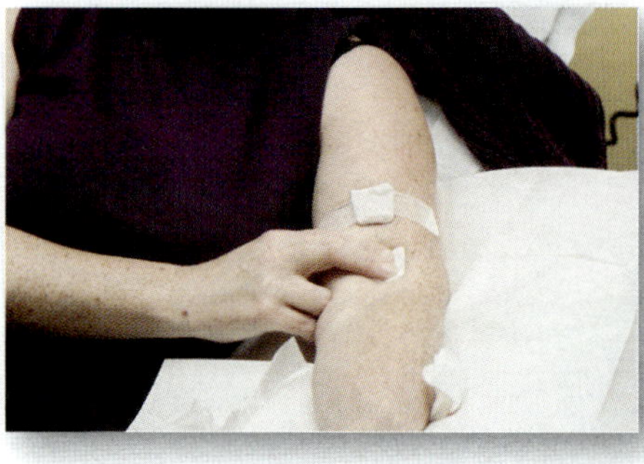

7 The needles are removed at the end of the dialysis session.

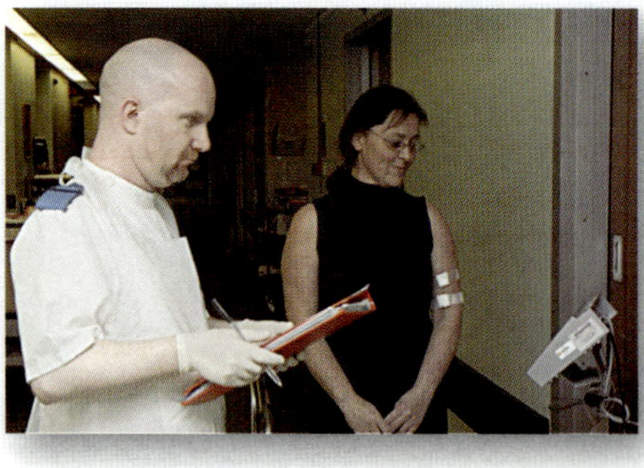

8 Her weight and blood pressure are checked again.

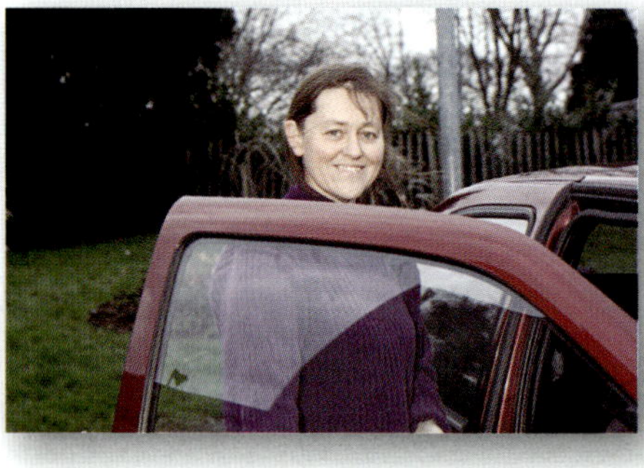

9 Patricia drives herself home. Some people need to use a hospital car or ambulance.

PD and haemodialysis – which is best?

Sometimes there are medical reasons why one type of dialysis is necessary. In many cases, though, the type of dialysis that will suit each person best can be chosen. This is not an easy decision, but the table shows some comparisons between dialysis types.

	PERITONEAL DIALYSIS	HAEMODIALYSIS
Where does dialysis happen?	At home	In hospital
What operation will I need?	Tube in tummy	Fistula in arm
How often does dialysis take place?	Four times a day (each treatment takes 20 minutes)	Three times a week, and treatment takes 5-7 hours in total, depending on travelling time
What are the main complications?	Tummy infection ('peritonitis') and problems with the dialysis tube in the tummy	Blood infection ('septicaemia') and problems with the fistula in the arm. Tiredness after each treatment
Is it painful?	Sometimes a little tummy pain	Local anaesthetic given before needles put into the arm
How strict are the fluid restrictions?	Quite strict	More strict
How strict is the diet?	Quite strict	More strict
Can I work?	Yes, but if on CAPD do exchange at lunchtime	Yes, may need evening or night dialysis if working a long day
Are holidays possible?	Yes, and quite easy. Either take fluid or have it delivered	Yes, but more difficult. Need to organise dialysis in another unit

Complications of dialysis

Unfortunately, all types of dialysis have complications. On haemodialysis or CAPD, about one third of people have no major complications, one third have occasional problems, and the remaining third have frequent problems. It is usually possible to switch between CAPD and haemodialysis if there are problems.

Deborah's story

Almost every female patient with whom I have spoken over the past 8 years – some like me, dealing with this condition in conjunction with other chronic conditions – has stated the single issue of their change in body image (both before and after transplantation) as being the most difficult to come to terms with. This is also an area in which little has been offered in the way of compromise.

There is little room for manoeuvre before transplantation with regard to the medical treatment of renal failure. But even pre-dialysis 'body image' is an issue, and the question of which of the two forms of dialysis to choose will impact on the female patient's perception of herself.

She needs to know in advance that, if she selects PD, she will have a distended stomach with a permanent plastic catheter protruding from its wall.
This makes being naked unattractive, and the implications of this need to be addressed frankly and fully.

By selecting haemodialysis she needs to know in advance that a fistula in her arm will be noticeable, will buzz (almost audibly) may become quite distended and will probably attract attention. Of course the bodily 'defects' both these forms bring about are almost reversible after a transplant.

Living with kidney failure

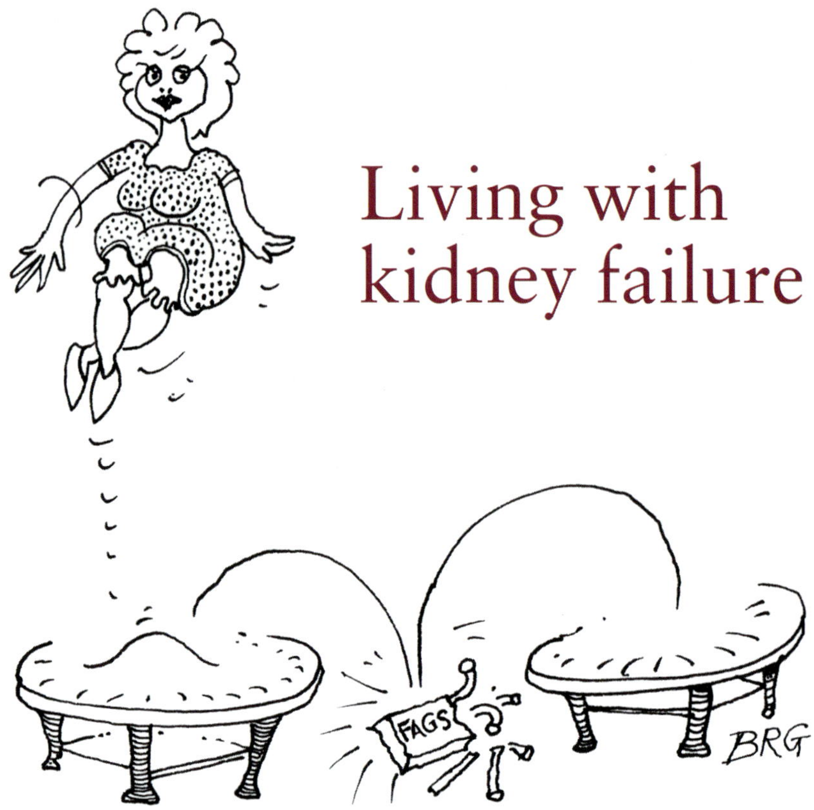

Smoking

Smoking tobacco carries a risk of damaging blood vessels and having a heart attack. Smoking also causes lung cancer.

Because kidney failure increases the risk of heart attacks and diseased blood vessels even in non-smokers, continuing to smoke with kidney failure carries an extremely high risk. Ask for help if necessary, because giving up an addiction to tobacco is not easy.

Exercise

General health benefits from regular exercise. This does not have to be vigorous – people should work to their limits while making a point of being active and mobile. This keeps muscle strength up, and helps the heart.

Some people find it helpful to take part in organised exercise at gyms or health clubs. Ask one of the doctors for advice before starting.

Holidays

People with kidney failure visit all parts of the globe. But do bear in mind that some remote places will have few facilities for dealing with kidney failure. Most of the world, though, has well-developed kidney failure services and can be visited quite safely.

Ask for advice well in advance of a holiday. Dialysis is provided free within the European Union. In other parts of the world, it may be necessary to pay for each haemodialysis session. Many Renal Units will pay for a limited number of sessions a year of holiday dialysis.

Up to date recommendations on vaccinations and other precautions such as malaria prevention are given on the Department of Health and British National Formulary websites. Advice on which vaccinations and drugs are suitable for kidney failure patients is given in the 'drugs' section of the Medical Information zone on the NKF website (see page 25 for website addresses). In some parts of the world, including India and the Middle East, there is a high incidence of hepatitis on dialysis units, and there may be a risk of catching one of these liver viruses.

Travel insurance should include cover for illnesses associated with kidney failure. Not declaring kidney failure to an insurance company may result in cheaper insurance, but there may be no cover for a serious illness or accident, as this would usually have some effect on the kidneys. Although emergency medical care is provided in the European Union under the E111 system, this does not provide free treatment in all countries, and does not cover important care such as an air ambulance to get home, so some insurance even when in the European Union is advisable. Advice on E111 cover is given by the Department of Health (see website on page 25) and in the booklet available with the form from post offices.

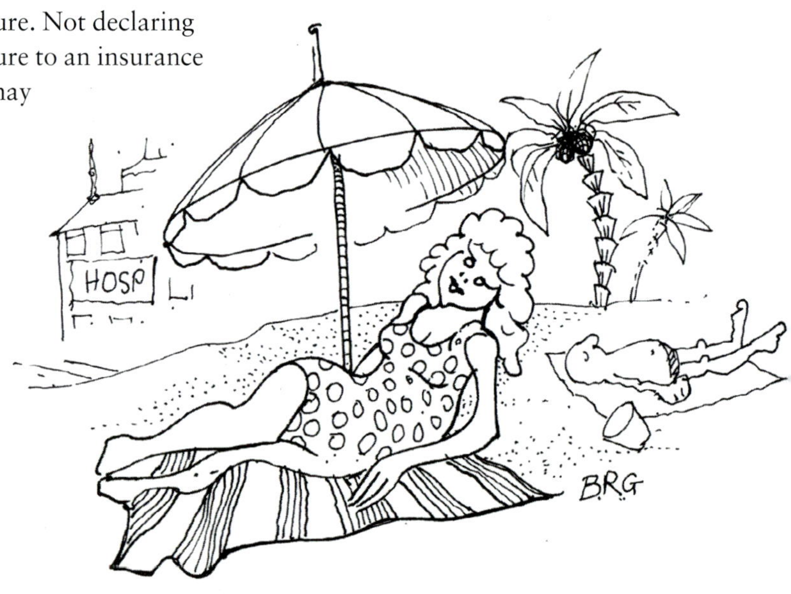

Sex

Sexual problems are common for men and women who have kidney failure. Not only are emotional problems more likely to occur, but also there are a number of medical conditions that can affect sexual function, in both men and women. Research has shown that people of all ages may have sexual problems, but these are more frequent in the mid-40s and later.

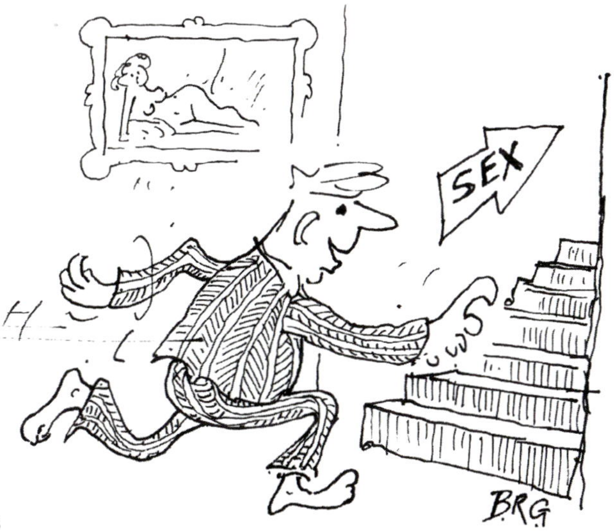

Some people worry that sex may not be possible when they are receiving dialysis treatment, especially peritoneal dialysis where they have a tube in the tummy. They can be reassured, however, that this need not stop them from having an enjoyable love life.

Sexual problems are made worse by anaemia, and treatment with EPO may help some people. Problems with getting or sustaining an erection in men may be treated with Viagra® or other similar drugs. More information on addressing sexual problems for both men and women can be found on the NKF website (see 'Other sources of help and advice' on page 25 for details).

Although many individual doctors are uncomfortable about giving advice about sexual problems, most kidney units have access to a local specialist, so it is helpful to ask one of the doctors or nurses to make a referral. In some areas, however, there may be rather a long wait.

Sexually transmitted diseases can occur in people with kidney failure in just the same way as in other people so, unless you are confident your relationship is stable and monogamous, do make sure you use a condom. Practice safe sex!

Having babies

Kidney failure reduces fertility, particularly in women. Men are likely to have a reduced sperm count, but are still able to father children at any stage. By contrast, women who are on dialysis often stop ovulating; but this is not always the case, so proper means of contraception should be used too. Pregnancy on dialysis is difficult, can be complicated, and only rarely results in a healthy baby born at the right time. It is usually possible for women with early kidney disease, but the risks to both mother and baby will be higher than usual. It is important women discuss their intentions with their doctor, before getting pregnant, if they plan to have a family.

Women who have had a kidney transplant are in a much better position to become pregnant and give birth to a healthy baby. However, this is not without risk either so it is important to talk to your doctor first if you have a transplant and wish to try for a baby. Use contraception at all stages unless you are sure that pregnancy is both safe and what you want.

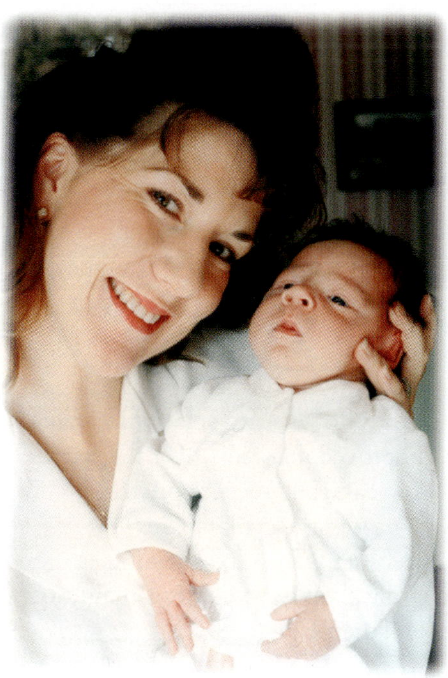

Sarah and baby George. Sarah's father gave her a transplant ten years ago.

Deborah's story

The issue of having children is also affected by renal failure. I know of many healthy children successfully conceived post-transplant, and indeed of many healthy children carried into early stage renal failure.

I do believe that my inability to sustain a successful pregnancy is directly attributable to years of nerve damage in diabetes followed by renal failure. This is an area of great regret for me and I believe deprived me of exploring a side of me that is quintessentially 'female'. This then is another area a woman will need to address in the early stages of renal failure. She needs to be clear on where she stands on these issues and be made aware of what opportunities are available to her for her future.

Work

Many people with kidney failure are in full-time work, and have better sickness records than their 'healthy' friends. Most employers are very helpful to their employees with kidney failure, but may be concerned at first. Staff at your Renal Unit can write reports for your occupational health department at your place of work.

Insurance and mortgages

Kidney failure has to be declared for most new mortgage applications and life or employment insurance policies. Provided you are generally fit apart from kidney failure, it should be possible to get a mortgage or insurance but a report from the specialist is often required. If there are problems getting a policy, ask for advice from your local kidney patients' association or the NKF as there are brokers and companies who are used to helping people with kidney failure.

Deborah reflects

A woman having dealt with the time spent in renal failure, followed by the period surrounding a transplant and all that that journey entails, will still be left with the burning question of how much to tell people about her 'condition' and, more importantly, when. For my part, the moment I am within a 'medical' environment I am happy to tell all. Outside of this I have got it so wrong too many times to venture an opinion on how to deal with specifics in this issue. Suffice to say it is very easy to become a 'medical bore' and to put people off their food!

I guess that maintaining links with good friends throughout renal failure is vital for several reasons. For a start it eliminates a large part of the problem of how much of your 'history' is required in order for people to gain an opinion of you; and it gives a fairly accurate indicator of how much involvement the people closest to you want.

Talking to fellow (single) female transplant recipients it has dawned on me that we appear to have acquired an unrealistic 'this is my problem and I don't expect anyone else to deal with it' approach to our future. That's a shame because life is too short and everyone has their own form of 'baggage'. Everybody is a product of how they have dealt with what life has thrown at them. To conquer renal failure and live with transplanted organs has got to be a source of admiration!

How long will someone with kidney failure live?

How long someone will live when they have kidney failure depends on problems in the heart and other parts of the body, as well as on the success of the dialysis or transplant. Each of these factors varies from person to person and an individual assessment needs to be made. Even then, it is not possible to predict anyone's survival accurately. Indeed, many people will die from other causes entirely.

Some people who develop disabling or painful conditions ask to have their dialysis stopped. Death from kidney failure then takes place in 1-3 weeks. Any sickness or agitation can be treated with drugs. Stopping dialysis is clearly a major and irreversible decision, but is not illegal or regarded as a form of suicide. The renal team will discuss the motives someone might have for stopping dialysis, but will support anyone who makes this difficult decision.

The outlook for people on dialysis and following transplantation has improved markedly over the last 20 years, and recent updated statistics are available on the websites for United Kingdom Transplant (**www.uktransplant.org**) and the Renal Registry (**www.renalreg.com**). The average survival four years after starting dialysis in people aged 45-64 years is about 70 %, though this tends to be better for younger patients (80% in those below the age of 40) and not quite as good for those in the older age bracket (going as low as 25% for people aged 80 or over). These figures have been compiled by the Renal Registry. A successful transplant increases survival compared to dialysis. However these are only average figures. You are an individual – you are not average.

Jargon busting

Acute Short-term and of rapid onset, usually requiring a rapid response.

Anaemia A shortage of red blood cells in the body, causing tiredness, shortage of breath and pale skin. Anaemia is measured by the haemoglobin level (see below).

APD Abbreviation for automated peritoneal dialysis – a form of peritoneal dialysis that uses a machine to drain the dialysis fluid out of the person and replace it with fresh solution. APD is usually carried out overnight while the person sleeps.

Arteries Blood vessels that carry blood from the heart to the rest of the body.

BP Abbreviation for blood pressure.

CAPD Abbreviation for continuous ambulatory peritoneal dialysis. A continuous form of PD in which a person performs the exchanges of dialysis fluid by hand. The fluid is usually exchanged four times during the day, and is left inside the person's body overnight.

Catheter A flexible plastic tube used to enter the interior of the body. Different types of catheter may be used for haemodialysis, peritoneal dialysis or to drain urine from the bladder.

Cells The tiny units from which all living things are built up. Cells in different parts of the body look different from each other and perform different functions (for example, skin cells are very different from blood cells).

Chronic Long-term and of slow onset, not usually requiring immediate action.

CKD An abbreviation for 'chronic kidney disease'. This includes both chronic kidney failure and milder forms of kidney disease.

Clearance The removal of the toxic waste products of food from the body. Clearance is one of the two main functions of the kidneys. In kidney failure, clearance is inadequate and toxins from food build up in the blood.

Creatinine A waste substance produced by the muscles when they are used. The higher the blood creatinine level, the worse the kidneys (or dialysis or a kidney transplant) are working.

CRF Abbreviation for 'chronic renal failure', in which the kidneys are working at less than one third (30%) of normal.

Dialysis An artificial process by which the toxic waste products of food and excess water are removed from the body.

Diastolic blood pressure A blood pressure reading taken when the heart is relaxed. It is taken after the systolic blood pressure and is the second figure in a blood pressure measurement.

Donor A person who donates (gives) an organ to another person (the recipient).

End-stage renal failure (ESRF) A term for advanced chronic kidney failure. People who develop ESRF will die within a few weeks unless they are treated by dialysis or transplantation. These treatments control ESRF but cannot cure it.

EPO Abbreviation for erythropoeitin.

Erythropoeitin A hormone made by the kidneys, which stimulates the bone marrow to produce red blood cells.

Established renal failure (ERF) Another term for end stage renal failure or ESRF.

Fistula An enlarged vein, usually at the wrist or elbow, that gives access to the bloodstream for haemodialysis. The fistula is created by a surgeon in a small operation. This increases the flow of blood through the vein and causes it to enlarge, making it suitable for haemodialysis needles.

Haemodialysis A form of dialysis in which the blood is cleaned outside the body, in a machine called a dialysis machine or kidney machine. Each dialysis session lasts for three to five hours, and sessions are usually needed three times a week.

Haemoglobin (Hb) A substance in red blood cells that carries oxygen around the body. Blood levels of haemoglobin are measured to look for anaemia. A low Hb level indicates anaemia.

Hormones Substances that act as chemical messengers in the body. Hormones travel around the body in the blood and control how other parts of the body work.

Hypertension High Blood Pressure

Kidneys The two bean-shaped body organs where urine is made. They are located at the back of the body, below the ribs.

mmol/l Abbreviation for millimoles per litre. A unit used to measure the blood levels of many substances. Creatinine is measured in smaller units called micromoles per litre (μmol/l).

Nephrology The study of the kidneys.

PD Abbreviation for peritoneal dialysis.

Peritoneal cavity The area between the two layers of the peritoneum inside the tummy. The peritoneal cavity contains the abdominal organs, including the stomach, liver and bowels. It normally contains only about 100 ml of liquid, but expands easily to provide a reservoir for the dialysis fluid in peritoneal dialysis.

Peritonitis Inflammation of the peritoneum, caused by an infection. People on peritoneal dialysis risk getting peritonitis if they touch the connection between their PD catheter and the bags of dialysis fluid. Most attacks are easily treated with antibiotic drugs.

Phosphate A mineral that helps calcium to strengthen the bones. Phosphate is obtained from foods such as dairy products, nuts and meat. In kidney failure, phosphate tends to build up in the blood.

Potassium A mineral that is normally present in the blood, and which is measured in the biochemistry blood test. Either too much or too little potassium can be dangerous, causing the heart to stop.

Recipient In the context of transplantation, a person who receives an organ from another person (the donor).

Red blood cells Cells in the blood which carry oxygen from the lungs around the body.

Renal Relating to the kidneys.

Satellite haemodialysis unit A place where some patients go for haemodialysis away from the main hospital renal unit. These units tend to be more friendly and less frantic than most main hospital buildings.

Sodium A mineral that is normally present in the blood that comes from salt (sodium chloride), and which is measured in the biochemistry blood test.

Systolic blood pressure A blood pressure reading taken when the heart squeezes as it beats. The systolic blood pressure is measured before the diastolic blood pressure and is the first figure in a blood pressure measurement.

Transplant kidney A kidney removed from one person (the donor) and given to another person (the recipient). Transplant kidneys may be either cadaveric transplants, living related transplants or living unrelated transplants.

Urine The liquid produced by the kidneys, consisting of the toxic waste products of food and the excess water from the blood.

Veins Blood vessels which carry blood from the body back to the heart.

Written information

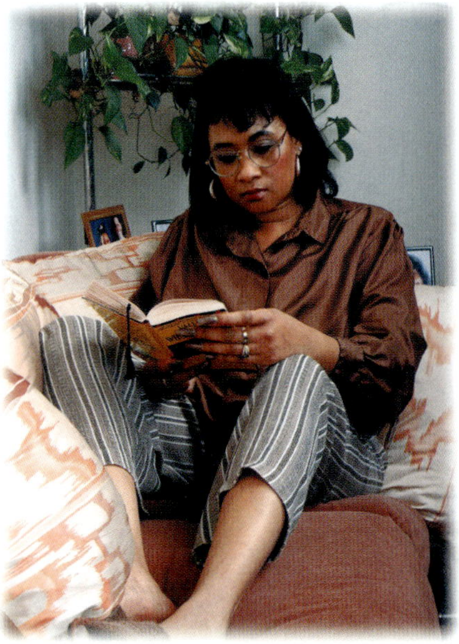

You will find many information leaflets on your Renal Unit, or from the National Kidney Federation.

The following books are also likely to be helpful:

Juliet Auer, *Living Well With Kidney Failure*. Class Publishing, 2004

Helena Jackson, Annie Cassidy and Gavin James, *Eating Well With Kidney Failure*. Class Publishing, 2005

Dr Andy Stein and Janet Wild, *Kidney Dialysis and Transplants: the 'at your fingertips' guide*. Class Publishing, 2002

Dr Andy Stein and Janet Wild, *Kidney Failure Explained*. Class Publishing, 2002

Dr Sarah Brewer, *Intimate Relations: living and loving in later life*. Age Concern Books, 2004

Dr Stewart A Cameron, *Kidney Failure: the facts*. OUP, 1996